The Ultimate Guide To:

Natural Remedies To Boost Energy Now!

Eliminate Fatigue, Stop Procrastination, And Achieve Anything With 25 Natural Remedies For Fatigue!

I0428309

Sarah Brooks

STOP!!! Before you read any further....Would you like to know the Secrets of Body Transformation?

If your answer is yes, then you are not alone. Thousands of people are looking for the secret to rapidly burn body fat, keep the weight off, become healthier, and truly transform their body and life for good.

If you have been searching for these answers without much luck, you are in the right place!

Not only will you gain incredible insight in this book, but because I want to make sure to give you as much value as possible, right now for a limited time you can get full **100% FREE access to a VIP bonus EBook** entitled **THE 7 KEYS TO BODY TRANSFORMATION!**

Just Go Here For Free Instant Access:

www.liveFitVIP.com

Legal Notice

Disclaimer Notice

Table Of Contents

Introduction

I want to thank you and congratulate you for purchasing the book, *"Natural Remedies To Boost Energy Now!: The Ultimate Guide To Natural Remedies For Energy! - Eliminate Fatigue, Stop Procrastination, And Achieve Anything With 25 Natural Remedies For Fatigue!"*

This book contains proven steps and strategies on how to live a more energetic and exciting life! Best of all the strategies in this book don't rely on typical ways to boost energy, such as caffeine or other harmful stimulants.

Instead of relying on those substances, you'd soon be carrying out techniques that provide vigor despite being simple, safe, and effective – some merely involve a glass of water. Are you excited? Well, it's no surprise that you are.

Thanks again for purchasing this book, I hope you enjoy it!

Chapter 1 – Superior Beverages Choices

Are you a slave to coffee's stimulating power? Are you among those who've already spent a fortune on energy drinks? Maybe you're allergic to caffeine (or any other kind of pick-me-up substance), and that's why you're looking for an alternative. Well, whatever your reason might be, you're about to discover 25 excellent ways to fight tiredness.

Here's the first one – drink a glass of cold water. It's alright if you're a bit skeptical of this suggestion, though. After all, it does seem too simple to provide any noteworthy benefit. However, you should keep in mind that low temperatures have a blood-rushing effect – when cold water passes through the body, the entire circulatory system speeds up its key processes.

So, what happens when blood flows faster (particularly to vital organs)? The body enters a state of alertness (since it's essentially protecting itself from the sudden drop in warmth), which in turn means that the mind would immediately be rid of any thought related to sleep. If you're really running out of energy though, then you might want to rely on a technique that involves sugar.

As you might have expected, the second fatigue-fighting technique is simply drinking a sugar-and-water solution. You're probably thinking of one question right now – isn't sugar a stimulant like caffeine? Truth be told, it isn't – lots of people just assume that it is. After all, kids who eat sweets by the handful cause all sorts of mischief (in other words, they experience periods of hyperactivity).

How does sugar boost alertness then? Well, there are two answers to that. The first one pertains to the sweet granule's energy-rich nature, as well as its structural simplicity. In other words, whenever you drink a sugar-and-water concoction, your body gets an almost immediate increase in energy since it doesn't have to process sugar as much as other vigor-giving substances.

Aside from giving you calories to burn, a sugar-and-water beverage also increases the amount of insulin in your body. To explain a bit further, whenever the body detects that sugar is becoming abundant, it produces more insulin so that sugar levels would go down quickly enough. Insulin has a useful "side effect" though – whenever more of it is available, the brain ends up being stimulated.

If you're not too keen on drinking plain sugar water, then you might want to rely on this tiredness buster – adding lemon juice (or a few slices of the fruit) to a glass of water. Lemon – no matter how sour it is – still contains sugar. It isn't the same as table sugar though, especially since fruit sugar (which experts call fructose) doesn't usually hasten the insulin production process.

Even though lemon water does provide the body with additional energy, it doesn't have as much calories as its table-sugar-containing counterpart. So, is adding fruit juice to H_2O just a poor (but a bit more diabetic-friendly) alternative to mixing sugar and water together? The answer's no. Lemon has an innate sourness that makes it a potent pick-me-up.

After reading that, you might think that drinking extremely sour lemon water is a perfect way of battling sleepiness. That might be a good course of action from time to time, but you shouldn't turn it into a regular habit. If you're wondering why, then you should keep this in mind – anything that's sour can lead to increased gastritis susceptibility and also worsen ulcer-related pain.

Is there a beverage that's suited for someone who doesn't like drinking cold water but has both diabetes and tummy issues? Well, there is – soymilk. It should be pointed out right away though, that the vegan alternative to fresh cow's milk contains moderate amounts of purine – a substance that's linked to both insulin issues and joint concerns.

Simply put, it wouldn't be wise to drink a glass of soymilk every time you feel tired. Drinking a single glass a day should be enough if you have any medical condition that's associated with uric acid. If you're perfectly healthy and you're not getting a lot of purines from the other parts of your diet, then two to three glasses should be fine.

While you're already aware that soymilk isn't something that you should enjoy throughout the entire day, you still don't know how it eliminates the feeling of fatigue. The sheer abundance of Vitamin B12 makes the beverage an excellent alternative to stimulant-containing drinks. That's right; sleepiness is sometimes a sign of Vitamin B12 deficiency.

Is there an alternative to soymilk that's slightly tastier? Even lemon water doesn't taste that great, right? Actually, if you'd add fruits to an ordinary protein shake, then you'd have something that contains both energy-rich carbohydrates and B Vitamins. Since the kind of fruit that you'd add depends on your preferences, you won't have any flavor-related dilemma.

Here's what you must know though – you shouldn't skip the add-on. Even if you're feeling adventurous enough to drink unflavored protein shake (or you simply want to have a lower-calorie beverage), you still need to add a few slices of fruit so that the B Vitamins that you'd get would really be useful. After all, those nutrients mainly hasten the conversion of food to energy.

Just to help you even further, here are several suggestions on which fruits could make your energy-booting beverage much more potent – strawberry (this fruit isn't merely good for the eyes, it's also rich in metabolism-accelerating Vitamin C), banana (a superb, nutritionally-diverse choice for people with digestive issues), and blueberry (known to enhance both mental focus and memory).

Chapter 2 – Body Movements For Increased Energy

At this point, you've already learned about five top-notch ways of staying awake. It's likely though, that you still haven't found a tiredness solution that suits you. If you like to move a lot, then these exercises should be perfect for you. Yes, physical activity does make your mind more alert, especially since movement prevents thoughts of sleep from popping up.

Here's one kind of exercise that doesn't require too much effort – walking in place. A minute's worth of walking (regardless of how quick your pace is) is often enough to shock the brain into heightening its alertness. What's so good about this simple workout is that you don't even have to move somewhere spacious. You could even do it in front of your desk while you're in the office.

If walking gave you a quick energy boost, then jogging (or even running) in place should be a much better option. However, you have to remember that the latter is slightly more tiring than the former – even though jogging in place might be able to give you a temporary boost in energy, doing it for far too long could result in sudden naptimes. Usually, a half-a-minute session is more than sufficient.

There are instances in which standing up isn't even an option. Well, you shouldn't worry since there are pick-me-up routines that could be done while sitting. Leg lifts are excellent examples of those while-seated exercises. If you're wondering whether it's difficult, then just think about this – the activity simply requires you to lift your legs, one after the other, about twenty times.

While leg lifts are definitely a lot safer than most other exercises, you still need to follow a few precautionary reminders. For one, you have to check whether your seat is sturdy enough to support your weight (particularly while you move). Aside from that, you mustn't keep your body lifted (with your arms) while raising your legs – even though that seems fun, your shoulders (or the chair) might give out.

If you know for a fact that your body is the very definition of strength, and you're quite confident that your seat wouldn't break even if it isn't used in the normal way, then you might want to try doing body lifts. Just hold on to your chair's armrests and try to lift your entire body upwards. After you've reached the maximum height, move back down slowly.

How many repetitions of that up-and-down movement should you do? There's no specific answer to that, but since you're trying to fight sleepiness and you don't want to feel even more tired, then you shouldn't go past 10 counts. It might even be better if you wouldn't exceed the 15-second mark (especially if you could only lift your body slowly).

If you prefer workouts that are much more engaging and you don't have space-limitation issues, then you might want to try doing some jumping jacks. Simply jump and move your feet apart while you're moving your arms right above your head (your palms should touch one another). Once you land and you're in that feet-apart, hands-together position, jump back into the normal standing stance.

Upright leg curls are superb substitutes to jumping jacks. To benefit from upright leg curling, all you need to do is to stand with your feet apart (bend your knees slightly) and then lift one of your legs behind you. Move that leg back down, and begin to raise the other leg. In short, just repeat the moving-back-down motion for one leg as you transition into lifting the other.

Ten seconds' worth of either jumping jacks or standing leg curls should be sufficient to convince your mind and body that they need to stay alert (and burn more calories to keep you awake). It's vital to remind you though, that you have to stretch before and after doing those exercises no matter how brief they might be. If you don't, then you might experience aches and even suffer from injuries.

Chapter 3 – Mental Stimulation To Boost Energy

So far, you've discovered 11 different tiredness busters. However, you haven't learned anything about activities that directly (and solely) stimulate the mind. Here's one example of those mental pursuits – think of your goals. What kind of goals should you focus your mind on? Well, anything should be fine – it doesn't matter whether you ponder upon the long term or the short term.

If you start thinking of things that could make you worry or upset you (the opportunities that you've missed in the past for example), then you must refocus your thoughts towards the positive. Elevated blood pressure and tiredness are linked after all, and the last thing that you'd want to happen is to suffer from stroke or heart attack while trying to stay awake.

As you know by now, beating fatigue is often as easy as keeping the mind occupied and preventing it from thinking about sleep. That's why it's also advantageous to play videogames whenever you feel too tired. It's best to point out though, that some types of videogames are much better "stimulants" than the others.

First-person shooters (titles that essentially give you a gun and let you fire away on all sorts of baddies) and arcade-style racers (games that make you forget about car physics and traffic rules) are two excellent choices. A role-playing game (which usually let you explore a virtual world) would also be a good pick, as long as it offers quick bursts of action.

If you're not interested in videogames and you don't intend to try playing them in the near future, then you might want to go a classic route. In other words, you should challenge someone to 30-second guessing game (or a whole minute if you'd like to take turns). Whether you're the one guessing or you're the "quizmaster", you're bound to feel energized.

Did you say that everyone around you is too serious to play a game? That shouldn't be a problem at all. Instead of trying to convince others to take part in your guess-what challenge, simply strike a conversation. It's almost impossible for your mind to fall asleep (no matter how tired you are) while you're talking to someone, especially if the conversation's about something controversial.

Are you worried that you'd pick a bad topic? Well, these should be interesting to almost anyone – animal testing (a debate between human safety and animal rights), human trafficking (why it still exists despite the fact that society has already changed so much), and the global war on terror (whether it actually protects people or it's merely a way to give governments greater control).

Aside from playing games and engaging in conversations, you could also get a fee pep talk. That doesn't mean that you need to look for a person who's willing to encourage you (verbally). All you have to do is to get a device that has access to the web, and afterwards visit your favorite video-sharing website. Look for the site's search bar, key in "free pep talk", and press enter.

Soon enough, you'd be looking at a results page that's linked to hundreds and even thousands of inspirational videos. If the sheer number of motivational clips is a bit off-putting to you, then you shouldn't close that browser. You just have to make your search much more specific using longer word strings – "free pep talk study", "free pep talk career", and "free pep talk life" are a few good examples.

By the way, these mental stimulation strategies are easier to carry out than most other energy-boosting techniques. Unlike workouts for example, these fatigue-fighting methods don't come with the overexertion downsides. That means that it's unlikely to feel even more tired after doing several mind-focused activities. So, don't be afraid to mix and match what you've discovered in this chapter.

Chapter 4 – Outside Forces Robbing Your Energy

Right now, you already know 16 different ways to combat sleepiness. This chapter contains five additional techniques that might prove to be much more useful than those already discussed – that is, if you have the option to "change" your environment. After all, tiredness is sometimes triggered by the sleep-inducing nature of certain places.

What kinds of locations make people sleepy? You're thinking about that question, right? Well, warm places tend to make the body feel relaxed, and thus they make it harder to stay awake. Rooms that are dimly lit could also make a person think about slumber since the lack of bright lights simulates nighttime darkness. Silence-filled quarters also intensify the yearning for sleep.

After becoming aware of those facts, you've probably thought about places that could have a stimulating effect on tired minds and bodies. Have you considered the park? Parks that have lots of people tend to have an invigorating impact – particularly due to the sheer amount of things that are happening within such recreational areas (the mind finds it difficult not to observe).

If the park near your place is the very definition of tranquility, then you might want to find another energy-giving spot. If you could go to a room that's covered in warm-colored paint, then you might just be able to beat tiredness. Colors that are usually described as visually intense (such as red) are more than capable of grabbing the mind's attention for long periods.

What's so good about that suggestion is that it highlights the possibility of creating your very own power area. In other words, you could choose one part of your home and make its walls much warmer to the eye (through painting, of course). If you often spend time in the office, then you might want to tell your superior about the benefits of warm colors.

Here's another method of battling tiredness – stay near the air conditioner. As you've read a while back (in the first chapter), low temperatures make the body a lot more active internally. So, if ever you'd choose to sit right beside the AC, your body wouldn't be able to prioritize relaxation; instead, it'd be busy protecting your organs from the cold.

There's no denying that some people really hate low temperatures. If you're among them, then you obviously prefer to go someplace warmer. As mentioned though, warmth has a relaxing effect. So, is there a workaround to that dilemma? There's actually one solution, but it'd only be useful if you live near nature – simply enjoy the sunny outdoors while standing.

Staying upright is a top-notch means of minimizing the sleep-inducing effect of warmth. The abundance of oxygen also keeps the mind alert and much more functional no matter how tired you might be – exhaustion is, in part, a sign of having insufficient amounts of oxygen. The sun keeps you awake as well, since it triggers Vitamin D production (yes, it's an energy-releasing nutrient).

Here's a location-related solution to fatigue that would surely suit you if you're in an urban neighborhood – go to the nearest shopping center. Much like parks, malls and marketplaces are often brimming with activity. Unlike parks though, shopping centers are much noisier – remember silence makes the mind focus on the wonders of slumber.

Aside from having various distracting sounds, those shop-filled places are equipped with bright lights. In short, malls and marketplaces represent the busyness of daytime (even at night), and your mind would never begin to think that it's time to sleep while you're in those establishments – not unless you're really running very low on energy and you've been awake for more than a day.

Chapter 5 –Nutrition Choices For Increased Energy

That's right, sometimes there's too much fatigue in your body. Should you use the previous 21 tips if you're at the brink of having a tiredness-induced breakdown? Simply put, you shouldn't – unless you're willing to risk your life just to stay awake (being truly productive is even out of the question). These four remaining strategies should help you avoid that kind of danger.

Here's the first (long-term) defense against sleepiness – eating the right way. Yes, your diet might actually be the reason why you're feeling less energetic as of late, especially if you're not getting the right amount of calories each day. So, the question now is this – what's the easiest way to determine your daily caloric needs? Well, you only have to look for calorie calculators online.

It should be pointed out though, that those web-based apps usually require two important pieces of info (aside from age and exercise level) – weight and height. Once you've identified the caloric sweet spot, you'd have to check your diet. Specifically, you must find out whether what you're eating provides you with enough energy – make adjustments if your diet just doesn't cut it.

While it's essential to monitor your caloric intake, you mustn't forget about one vital rule when it comes to eating – timing is the key. To be a bit more specific, you need to eat a lot during breakfast and go relatively moderate at lunch. It is fine if you're skeptical of that fatigue-fighting suggestion, but you should keep in mind that the digestive system also requires energy to function.

As you might have guessed after reading that, your body begins to feel relaxed (or even lethargic) right after you've enjoyed a big meal since most of your energy stores get burned to fuel the entire digestion process. While that effect might be fine early in the morning, it'd surely have a detrimental impact if it occurs after lunchtime (you should be productive during those hours, right?).

You should also ponder upon the amount of sleep that you've been getting. Teens need at least eight and a half hours of slumber every day. Adults, on the other hand, require less – seven hours is sufficient. It shouldn't be a surprise to you that sleep deprivation leads to much bigger alertness issues. After all, your mind and body wouldn't be able to refresh and regenerate themselves.

If you're not convinced of the importance of sleep (and it's link to mental clarity and attentiveness), then you should think about this fact – in the United States alone, roughly a hundred thousand motor vehicle accidents each year are caused by drowsiness – a key sign of sleep deprivation. By the way, more than a thousand of those accidents lead to fatalities.

What's the 25th long-term sleepiness-busting technique? It's actually exercise. Not the kind that you've read about in the second chapter. This is all about moderately lengthy ones that are done on a regular basis. Brisk walking for half an hour each day is a great example of those fitness-boosting activities. Of course, following a workout video works too.

Why's fitness a vital part of the battle against tiredness? Truth be told, people with the right body-mass index use energy at a much more efficient pace than those classified as either overweight or obese. It's also crucial to note that the mind benefits from sufficient physical activity. Regular exercise is a top-notch way of convincing the brain to grow new cells after all.

Wait a minute. Do you know what the body-mass index is? It's a number that represents how much fat you have right now. In other words, it's a simple way of knowing whether you're fit or not. To determine your BMI, just use one of the many fitness calculators online – don't forget to compare the number that you'd get with the standard values though.

Finally, you've become much more knowledgeable on the matter of exhaustion, and you're aware that both short- and long-term solutions to the problem exist. All in all, you should now be able to stop tiredness in its tracks, as long as you remember that all sorts of things could trigger the problem and knowing the specific cause is crucial to pinpointing the best course of action.

Conclusion

Thank you again for purchasing this book on boosting energy!

I am extremely excited to pass this information along to you, and I am so happy that you now have read and can hopefully implement these strategies going forward.

I hope this book was able to help you understand that there are much healthier options out there to regain energy and banish tiredness.

The next step is to get started using this information and to hopefully live a happier, healthier and much more fulfilling life!

If you know of anyone else that could benefit from the information presented here please inform them of this book.

Finally, if you enjoyed this book and feel it has added value to your life in any way, please take the time to share your thoughts and post a review on Amazon. It'd be greatly appreciated!

Thank you and good luck!

Preview Of:

<u>Low Carb Diet</u>

Low Carb Diet Plan For Fat Loss For Life! Fast Acting Low Carb Diet To Lose Weight As Soon As Tomorrow!

Introduction

I want to thank you and congratulate you for purchasing the book, *"Low Carb Diet: Low Carb Diet Plan For Fat Loss For Life! Fast Acting Low Carb Diet To Lose Weight As Soon As Tomorrow!"*.

This book contains proven steps and strategies on how to get rid of excess weight fast!

So you have found yourself in the position of procrastination. You needed to start dieting months ago to get ready for that special event, or just to get ready to go to the beach or pool this year. Don't dismay you are not alone or too late. There are many proven strategies that can help you lose those extra pounds.

If you need to lose 10 lbs fast, drop a few inches to fit into that dress or maybe to fit into those favorite pants once again, then this book is exactly what you need. It will provide you with all the latest techniques and strategies to give you the surefire way to accomplish your desires in record time.

Don't wait any longer to have the body and health you have been missing out on. Many people wait for a perfect time to get in shape, lose a few pounds, and feel better about themselves, only to lose precious years in the process. The problem is that many times there isn't a perfect time to do anything in our lives.

The perfect time is NOW. If you really want something, there is no such thing as the wrong timing. Just take action now and you will soon be on your way to a much happier life.

Thanks again for purchasing this book, I hope you enjoy it!

Chapter 1: Faster Weight Loss Strategies

Slimming down does not necessarily mean you have to starve yourself. Provided the right diet and a proper exercise plan, it is not impossible to lose 10 pounds fast. So what does it exactly take to slim down fast enough? Below are some of the most important things you should keep in mind:

- Make complex carbs 30 percent of you calorie consumption

- Make protein 50 percent of your calorie intake

- Make healthy fats 20 percent of the total calories you eat

Avoid the common weight loss mistakes.

When it comes to losing the extra pounds, it is not only important that you learn the things you should be doing. It is equally crucial that you figure out the wrong things you may still be doing. A lot of people do weight loss mistakes without even knowing it. Little do they know what they think can slim them down are actually obstacles to their weight loss goals.

For instance, skipping meals is one of the most common practices. The plain truth is that it is an unhealthy practice. Some people also avoid dairy products altogether. But the fact is calcium contained in dairy products is helpful in burning calories and fat.

Water should not be avoided when dieting. Water can not only burn fat, it also helps the body get rid of toxins. Ice cold water for instance is very good because the body is forced to burn additional calories and fat to make sure the water you drink is properly heated to match your body temperature. You are also more than welcome to dose up on coconut water, fat free milk and other slimming drinks such as green tea, vegetable juice and yogurt based smoothies.

Stick to a healthy diet plan.

You have plenty of food options to include in your diet. The safest bet always includes raw fruits and vegetables. These healthy foods work not only to slim you down but also promote your overall health. These foods also give you energy to perform slimming exercises which can only increase the amount of weight loss.

Make time for exercise.

Dieting alone will not suffice. Cardiovascular exercises are recommended for overall weight loss. But there are targeted forms of workout too. Know your goal and implement the right type of exercise including the proper equipment for best results.

This all means you have to be ready to make changes on your lifestyle. A few sacrifices and compromises are called for here and there. But you know it is worth it when you start to get in a better shape.

Thanks for Previewing My Exciting Book Entitled:

"Low Carb Diet: Low Carb Diet Plan For Fat Loss For Life! Fast Acting Low Carb Diet To Lose Weight As Soon As Tomorrow!"

To purchase this book, simply go to the Amazon Kindle store and simply search:

"LOW CARB DIET"

Then just scroll down until you see my book. You will know it is mine because you will see my name "Sarah Brooks" underneath the title.

Alternatively, you can visit my author page on Amazon to see this book and other work I have done. Thanks so much, and please don't forget your free bonuses

DON'T LEAVE YET! - CHECK OUT YOUR FREE BONUSES BELOW!

Free Bonus Offer: Get Free Access To The www.LiveFitVIP.com VIP Newsletter!

Once you enter your email address you will immediately get free access to this awesome newsletter!

But wait, right now if you join now for free you will also get free access to the "The 7 Keys To Body Transformation" free EBook!

To claim both your FREE VIP NEWSLETTER MEMBERSHIP and your FREE BONUS eBook on THE 7 KEYS TO BODY TRANSFORMATION!

Just Go To:

www.liveFitVIP.com